H$_2$O Workouts®

Pool Pretzel

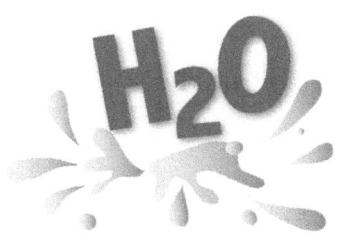

Francine Milford, LMT

Photographs by Paul, Larry and Francine Milford

ID: 978-1-105-83715-9

Caution
The techniques, ideas, and suggestions presented in this book are not intended as a substitute for proper medical advice. Any application of the techniques, ideas, and suggestions in this book is at the reader's sole discretion and risk. Please consult your health care provider before beginning this or any other exercise program.

Fitness for the Next Generation

As more people are recognizing the need to live healthier and better lives, they have begun to set goals on how they will achieve and maintain a healthy body through proper nutrition and balanced work schedules.

Before long, the entire face of a typical aerobic class was changed as millions of people attempted to find a way to add exercise into their daily lives. Classes ranged in levels from easy senior workouts and classes for pregnant women to the high paced, high intensity Boot Camp classes.

Soon, many people were experiencing injuries from pushing their bodies too long and too far. When people are impatient to see results, they tend to exercise for long hours in a short period of time. Overuse injuries are one of the most common injuries found in the fitness industry.

Now most facilities offer Tai Chi, Qigong, Yoga and Pilates for people who want a good workout without the stress and strain of strenuous exercise.

The Great Equalizer

I call the water environment, the Great Equalizer. When I have taught water aerobic classes I would have ladies enter the water on crutches and even one came to class in a wheelchair. Once in the water, you could not tell the ladies apart. In the water environment, everyone is equal and everyone can receive a workout that is right for them and their fitness level.

In this book I will be sure to list exercises in **LEVELS**. If you are a beginner, then please stick to **Level One** exercises. As your body becomes familiar with the moves and becomes stronger, then move on up to **Level Two** and **Level Three**. Remember, don't overdue your workouts or you risk injuring your body and not being able to exercise at all. I would rather see you do a short ten minute workout everyday to build yourself up to the half hour or hour workout.

Be sure to get the approval of your primary health care
physician before beginning this or any exercise routine.

Principles of Water Exercise

The water environment offers two important natural occurring effects to the water routine: buoyancy and resistance. Buoyancy is the property of being able to float. Buoyancy is also the power of a liquid to keep objects afloat; in this case, that object is you.

It is the natural ability of water to act as a cushion and in so doing, it protects you joints from injury, strain and re-injury. Many rehabilitation centers use the water environment in their treatment sessions.

While in the water environment, people can perform exercises they otherwise could not on land. Among these exercises are jumps, leaps, jumping jacks and pivots. Amazingly enough, the ability of water to be buoyant also allows water to provide resistance to water aerobics. Through changing direction, adding speed, or using longer levers, the water can provide a complete and thorough workout.

The water environment can become a natural total body workout. The more you put into your workout, the more you will receive from it. The faster you move, the harder the exercise becomes.

Water aerobics is also the perfect environment for those who are overweight or suffer from physical injuries. When you stand in water that is chest deep, you weigh only 10% of your normal body weight.

The water environment is also the great place to practice your golf or tennis swing. Even dancers and weight trainers can use the resistance in the water to build up muscles in a safe way.

Preparing to get Wet

When beginning your water exercise routine, the most important consideration is your swim suit. Find a suit that will cling comfortably to your body and still allow you freedom of movement.

Stay away from suits that will quickly fill with water with each jump that you take or that will ride up with each kick. If a suit isn't comfortable you will be fussing more with the suit than you will be concentrating on the exercises.

The second consideration is what to wear on your feet. Not everyone will be comfortable in wearing something on their feet while doing exercises in the water.

The bottom of the pool may be harsh on your feet through consistent movement. I haven't always had problems with this happening to my own feet, but it has happened, especially in backyard pools.

You have plenty of choices to make when selecting what to wear on your feet A pair of socks with good elastic is always an inexpensive purchase. I use a white booty sock that you will see later on in pictures in this book. I also own a pair of water socks (light shoes designed for walking in water) and a pair of water shoes. Yes, they actually look like tennis shoes but are made to go from land to water. I wear these shoes when I teach water aerobics as they add the perfect cushion for performing the moves on land.

There are also hand gloves, water buoys and pool noodles available to add resistance to your water workout. Many department stores and retail outlets now sell these products to water exercise enthusiasts. I highly suggest that you hold off on purchases until you have already begun your water workouts and find out whether or not you need more of resistance training, then make you purchase.

Tips for a Safe Workout

Do's and Dont's

- Do wear aqua shoes or aqua socks
- Do keep head in alignment of the spine.
- Do exercise in water that is of correct depth for you.
- Do relax and breathe slowly and deeply.
- Drink plenty of water before, during, and after exercising.
- Consult with your doctor before you begin exercising.
- Work at your own fitness level.
- Stop exercising if you feel faint, dizzy, nausea, or shortness of breath.
- Don't smoke or drink alcohol while exercising.
- Don't make fast, uncontrolled movements of the head or trunk in any direction.
- Don't use extreme range of motion.
- Don't use quick, jerky movement.
- Don't exercise with food or gum in your mouth.
- If you feel tired-stop

- For safety, there should be a lifeguard on duty during your workout or invite a friend to exercise with you.
- Never drink alcohol before, during, or immediately after a water workout.
- Perform your exercises in water that is chest high.
- Wait at least 1-3 hours after eating before working out
- When you enter the water that is cool, be sure to beginning walking, jogging, or bouncing right away to get your circulation moving.
- Always begin exercising slowly and then working up to more strenuous, energetic moves.
- Remember-Have fun!

Workout in Water

Warm-ups

As in any exercise program, it is important to prepare the body for the work that you are planning to put it through. We call this preparation, the Warm-Up.

In the Warm-Up you will increase the flow of blood to each and every muscle of the body. In this way, you will greatly reduce the risk of injury.

Warm-up exercises are usually gentle and slow activities that normally last 5 to 15 minutes. During this phase all the muscles and joints should be put through simple movements beginning with small range of motions and then increasing to larger, or full, range of motion.

In a typical land aerobic or workout class, we begin simply with marching in placing. The same holds true for water aerobics. In this chapter we will include several muscle groups that you will need to be sure you warm-up before beginning a water aerobics class. For some, this may be all the exercise that you can do in one day and if so, that is perfectly okay. What is important is move and stretch your body as often as you can throughout the day to keep it limber and lubricated.

When I received my certification in Aquatic Exercise, we practiced many types of water walking. Following a 3 to 5 minute warm-up exercise (such as marching in place) you could do some of the following walking exercises for the next 20-45 minutes:

- Walk forward and backwards
- Walk to the right and Walk to the left
- Walk in a big clockwise circle, then walk in a big counter-clockwise circle
- Walk on your toes

- Walk on your heels
- Walk like a crab sideways bouncing from flat feet with knees bent and open to the sides of your body.
- Walk forward and backward punching the water.
- Walk three steps and hop for one step.
- Do the Congo step in the water.
- Do the Bunny hop in the water.
- Do the Electric Slide in the water.
- Do your favorite Western Two Step in the water.
- Alternate between fast and slow walking to add intensity.
- Do the Soldier Walk, otherwise known on Goose Stepping
- Do Karate Kicks
- Walk doing knee lifts forward and front leg lift backwards
- Do Pendulum Swings with your legs side to side
- Do the Rocking Horse forward and backwards and change legs.
- Do Hamstring Curls forward and backwards.
- When stretching muscles in the warm-up phase it would be good if you could hold each stretch for at least 10 seconds (30 seconds is optimal).

Stretching

When performing the warm-up exercises and stretches, you should be able to feel slight warmth within your body. This is good and signals that you are preparing your body for the more vigorous workout that is to follow. The muscles that are stretched during the warm-up phase are the muscles that will be worked through the aerobic phase.

The Toe and Ankle Warm-ups

Some warm-up exercises and stretches can be performed inside, or at poolside, before you ever enter the water. If you find it difficult to spend more than 20 minutes in the water, then performing the warm-up stretches before entering the water may be a good idea. Remember, do the best that you can but don't push your body beyond its physical limitation and most of all – Have Fun!

1. Toes and Ankles

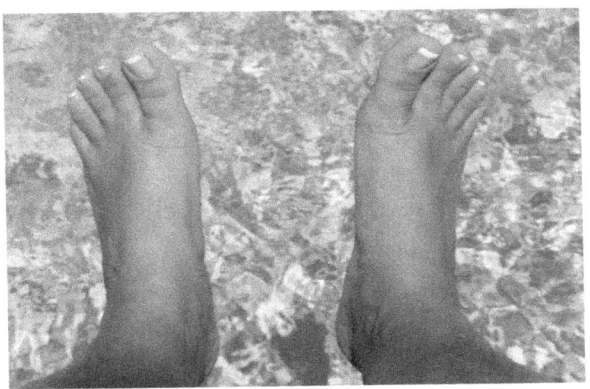

You can do this warm-up sitting in a chair before you enter the pool, or you may prefer to sit on the edge of the pool. Slowly point your toes towards you as far as you comfortably can, hold, and release. Do this exercise for a total of 8 repetiticns. Fee the stretch from each toe as your attempt to bring each toe towards you and then release it.

2.   Toes and Ankles

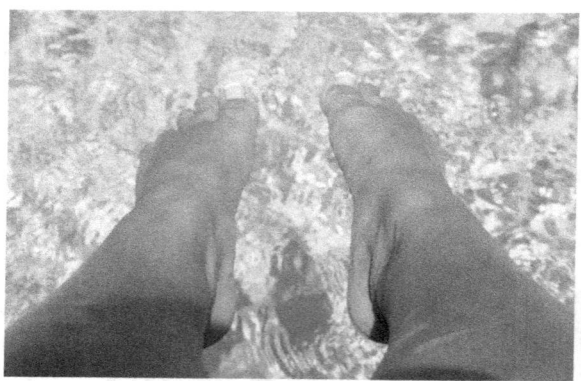

Press your toes away from your body, hold, and then relax the stretch. Perform this stretch for eight repetitions. Bring your focus to each of the toes and do not crunch them or fold them over one another. Allow each of the toes to enjoy and feel the stretch individually.

You will also be feeling a stretch in the front part of your leg, this is the anterior tibialis. When this muscle is not properly warmed up and stretched, many people suffer from Shin splints.

3. Toes and Ankles

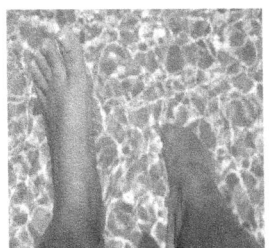 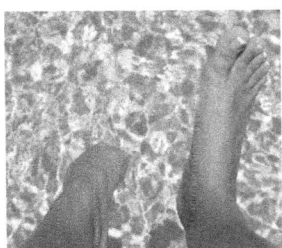

Alternate between flexing and extending your feet. Press your right toes away from your body while you bring your left toes toward you body, hold for a few seconds, and then relax the stretch. Now, bring your right towed toward your body and press your left toes away from your body at the same time. Continue for a total of eight repetitions.

If you are sitting poolside, you can perform this exercise either outside of the water, or inside of the warm. The choice is up to you.

4. Toes and Ankles

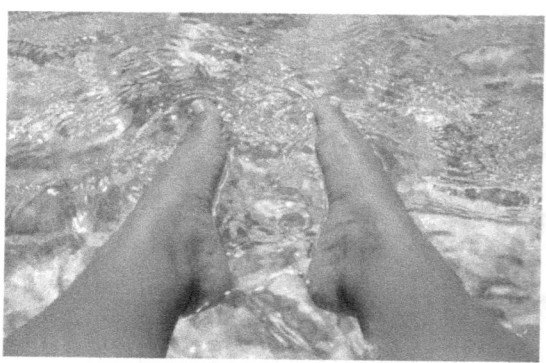

Press the soles of your feet towards each other, hold for a few seconds, and then relax the stretch. Perform this stretch for eight repetitions.

Now, press the soles of your feet away from each other. Repeat for a total of eight repetitions.

You will also be feeling a stretch in the front part of your leg, this is the anterior tibialis. The front of your leg should begin to feel warm, as well as, your ankles.

5. Toes and Ankles

Feet Swinging

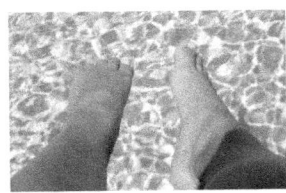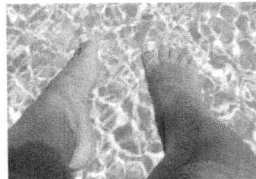

In the exercise above you will swing your feet to your right, hold for a few seconds, then swing your feet to the left, hold for a few seconds, and then relax. Perform these feet swinging exercises for eight repetitions.

Have fun with the exercise feeling the resistance of the water on your feet. Relax and enjoy.

6. Toes and Ankles

Circles

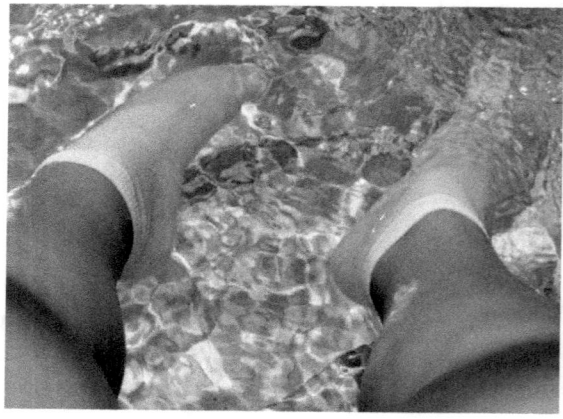

Using both feet at the same time, begin to move your feet in a circle clockwise. Begin by making eight small circles and then continue to enlarge each circle until you are making eight of the largest circles you can with you feet. Repeat the same exercise this time creating the smallest circles we can

Warm-ups for the Neck

Warm-ups for the neck can be performed on land before you enter the water environment. Do not push these stretches beyond what your physical capabilities are. Stretches should not be painful.

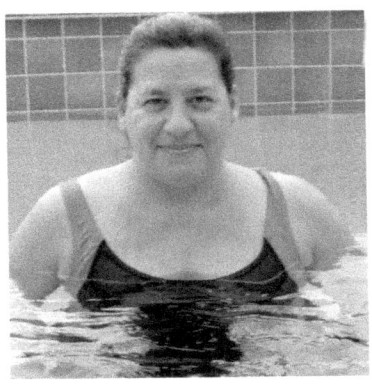

Starting Position

The starting point for the neck exercises will begin with the head in a neutral position as is shown in the diagram above, on the left. Keep you gaze in front of you at a slight angle downward. Be sure to breathe normally.

Neck Warm-ups

   1.   Neck

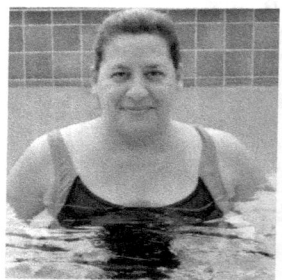 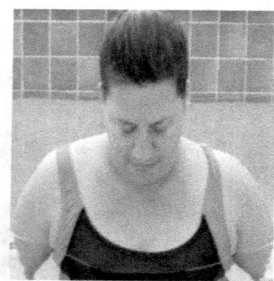

   With your head in the starting position take a nice deep slow breath in. As you exhale, slowly allow your head to fall forward touching your chin to your chest (note: if you cannot touch your chin to your chest, this is alright, don't force the movement.)

   Now, slowly inhale and begin to return your head to the starting position. Repeat this exercise for a total of eight repetitions.

2. Neck

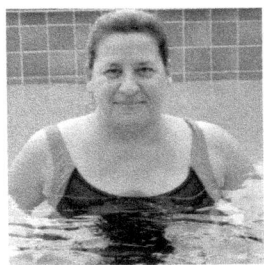 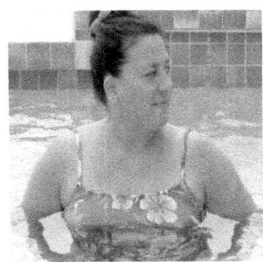

With your head in the starting position take a nice deep slow breath in. As you exhale, slowly turn your head to left aligning your chin to over your left shoulder. Now, slowly inhale and as you exhale, begin to return your head to the starting position.

With your head in the starting position take a nice deep slow breath in. As you exhale, slowly turn your head to right aligning your chin to over your right shoulder (note: if you cannot align your chin to over your shoulder, this is alright, don't force the movement.) Repeat this exercise for a total of eight repetitions.

3. Neck

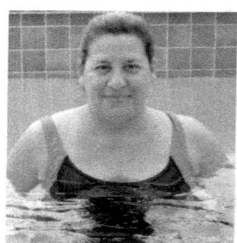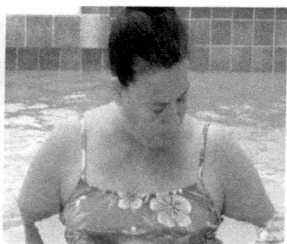

With your head in the starting position take a nice deep slow breath in. As you exhale, slowly allow your chin to drop to the left to a point that is located half way between the center of your chest and your left shoulder. Now, slowly inhale and as you exhale, begin to return your head to the starting position.

With your head in the starting position take a nice deep slow breath in. As you exhale, slowly allow your chin to drop to the right to a point that is located half way between the center of your chest and your right shoulder. Repeat this exercise for a total of eight repetitions.

4. Neck - Head Rolls

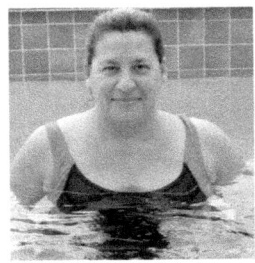 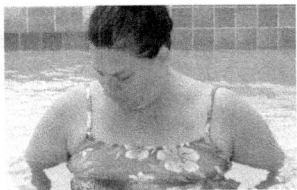

Imagine that your nose is like the hands of wall clock. The numbers of the wall clock are right in front of your face. Take a nice deep slow breath in and as you slowly exhale you will begin with your nose in the twelve o'clock position. Moving clockwise outline the numbers of the clock from 3, to 6, to 9, and ending back at the top at the number 12 position. Repeat for eight repetitions.

Now, repeat the above exercise, this time moving counter clockwise beginning at the 12 position moving down to the 9, 6, 3, and back to the top 12 position. Repeat for eight repetitions.

Warm-up for the Shoulders

1. Shoulders

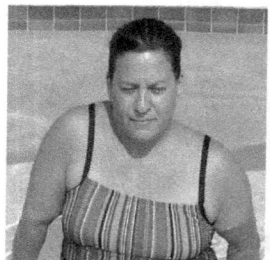 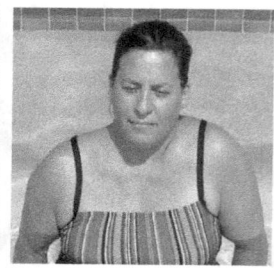

Bend your knees with your arms down at your sides. Inhale and bring your right shoulder up to your right ear and hold. As you exhale release the shoulder back down to starting position. Remember-do NOT bring your ear down to meet the shoulder. Repeat for a total of 8 repetitions. Repeat on the other side for a 8 repetitions.

You can also alternate between lifting right and left shoulders for a total of 16 repetitions.

2. Shoulders – Shrugs

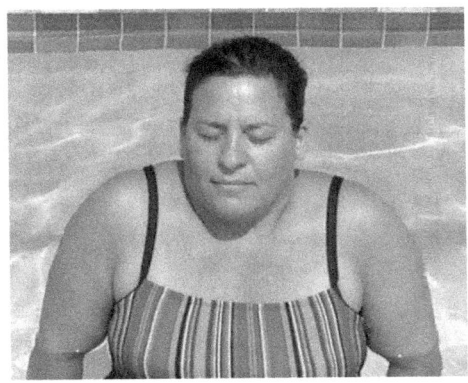

Inhale and bring both of your shoulders up to your ears and hold for a few seconds. As you exhale, allow both shoulders to relax and return to the starting position. Continue for a total of 16 repetitions.

This is a great exercise to do throughout the day to reduce stress.

3. Shoulders – Circles

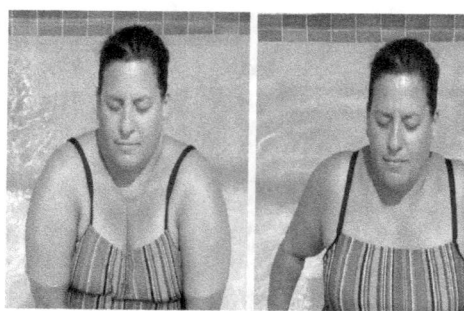

Inhale and bring both shoulders up to your ears and as you exhale allow the shoulders to push forward, then down, then back behind you forming a circle. As you inhale again pull the shoulders back up to your ears and repeat the circle of exhaling and allowing the shoulders to drop to the front, down to the sides and to the back before returning up to the ears again. Repeat for a total of eight repetitions.

Reverse the circles in the opposite directions for another eight repetitions.

Making the Noodle into a Pretzel

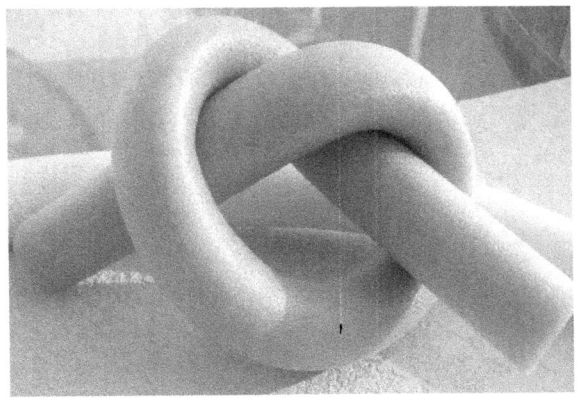

Making your pool noodle into a pretzel is easy and fun. Just fold both ends of the noodle into itself like you are going to tie a knot.

Try to make each end equal in length to help guarantee an equal workout. Don't worry; you will be able to undo the knot when you want to use your pool noodle again full length.

4. Arms and Shoulders

Starting Position

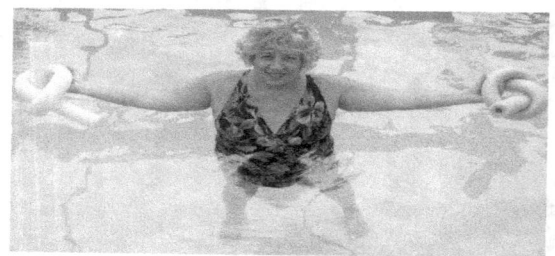

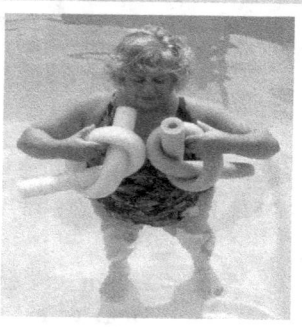

Place your hands on each of your pool pretzels. Inhale, and as you exhale bring your hands together in front of you. Hold and release to the starting position. Do for eight repetitions.

5. Arms and Shoulders

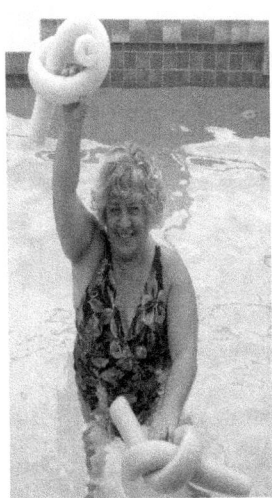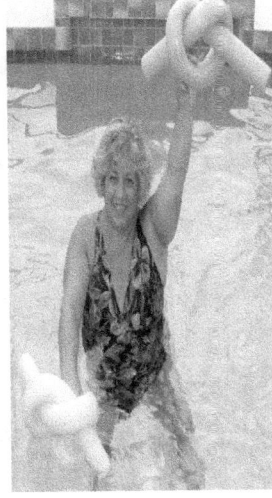

      With pool pretzels in each hand, place one hand in front of you while you raise the other hand over your head. Alternate your hands. Repeat for 8-16 repetitions.

6. Arms and Shoulders

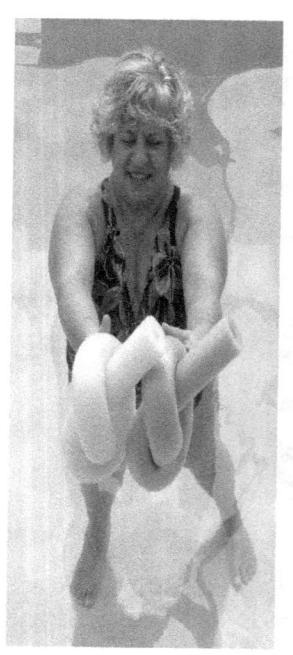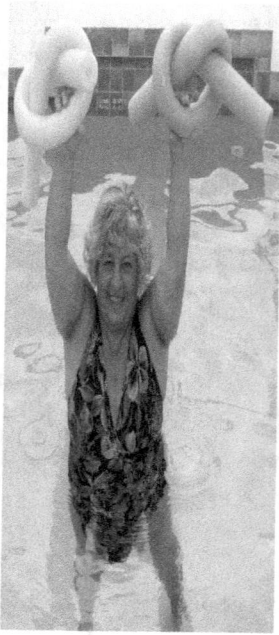

Place both pool pretzels in front of you and then raise them both at the same time over your head. Repeat for eight repetitions.

7. Arms and Shoulders

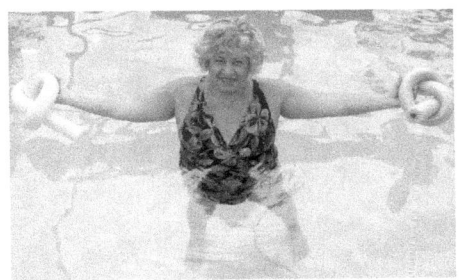

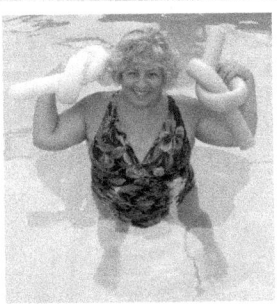

Extend your arms out to your side with palms facing upwards. Alternate bring both hands in towards your should at the same time. Repeat for a total of at least eight repetitions.

8. Arms and Shoulders

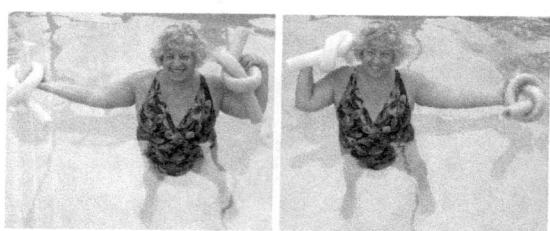

Extend your arms out to your side with palms facing upwards. Alternate bringing one hand in and touch your shoulder while extending the opposite hand. Switch hands and repeat this exercise. Repeat for a total of at least eight repetitions.

7. Arms and Shoulders

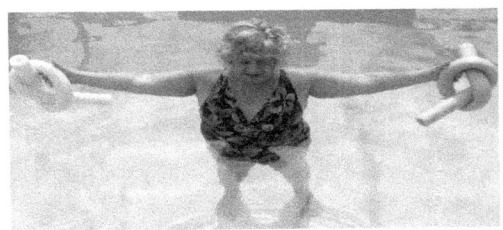

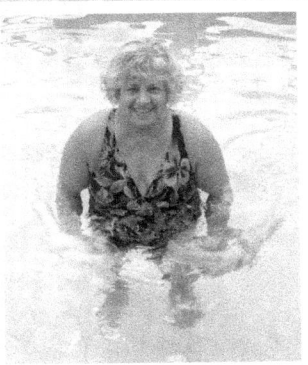

Place your arms out at your sides with palms facing forward and downward. Inhale and as you exhale bring your hands together in front of you in the water. Repeat for eight repetitions.

Back Stretch

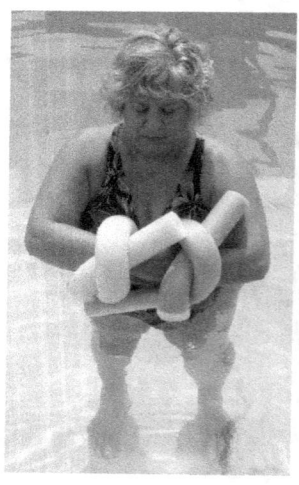 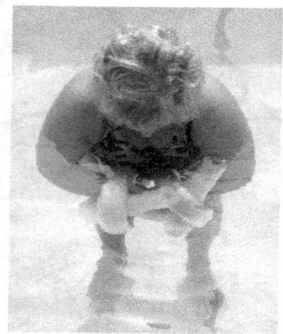

Stand with feet on the bottom of the
pool and knees slightly bent. Place both hands
inside of your pool pretzels. Take a deep breath
and as you exhale, press the hands down into the
water towards your lower abdomen. Hold and
release back to the starting position. Repeat for
eight repetitions.

**Note: If you feel any pain in your back with
this exercise, stop immediately.**

Deep End Workout

Place your pool pretzels on your upper arms as high up as you can place them. Now, enjoy some deep end workout exercises.

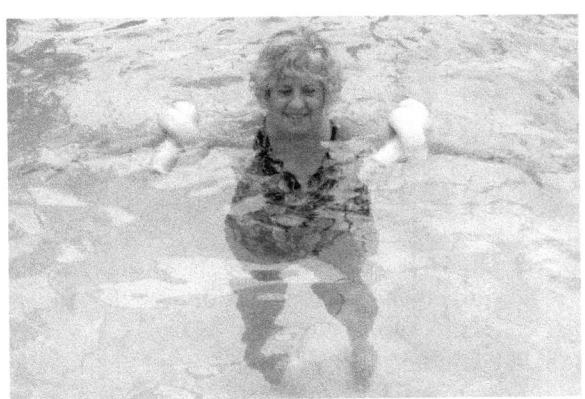

Starting Position

Let your legs daggle straight down towards the bottom of the pool. This is your starting position for several of the exercises that will follow.

Exercise One:

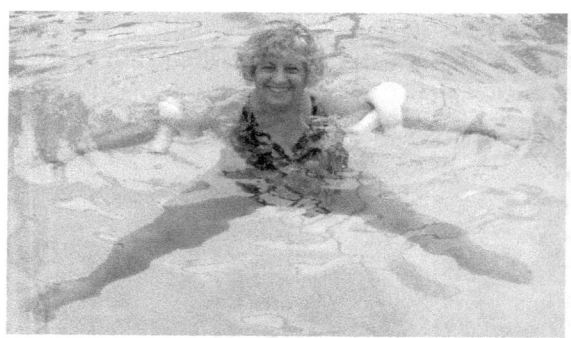

Level One-Let your legs daggle straight down towards the bottom of the pool. Inhale and as you exhale bring your legs out to your side. Inhale again and as you exhale, bring them back to center. Repeat for eight repetitions.

Level Two-When finished, turn around in the pool and face the opposite direction. Repeat the above exercises as listed in the exercise above.

.

Exercise Two:

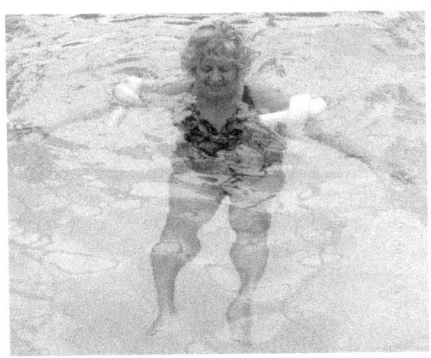

Let your legs daggle straight down towards the bottom of the pool. Inhale and as you exhale bring your legs out to the front of you together. Inhale again and as you exhale, bring them back to center. Repeat for a total of at least eight repetitions.

This stretch will add a nice stretch in through the muscles of the chest and abdominal area.

For a variation, with your legs together bring them straight back behind you as far as you can. Do not bend your knees. You can also alternate moving them forward and backward.

Exercise Three:

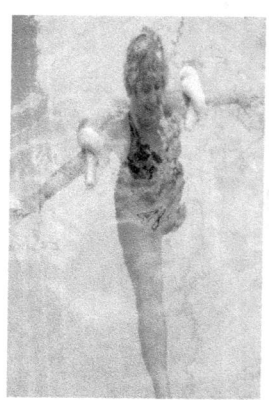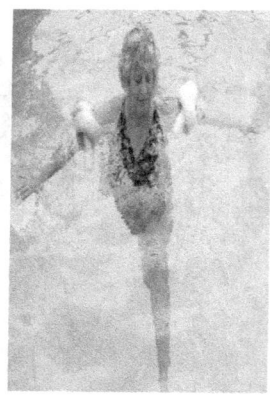

Let your legs daggle straight down towards the bottom of the pool. Inhale and as you exhale bring one leg straight out in front of you while bringing the other leg straight back behind them. Inhale again and as you exhale, bring them back to center. Repeat by switching legs. Repeat for a total of at least eight repetitions.

You can add intensity to this exercise by increasing speed.

Exercise Four:

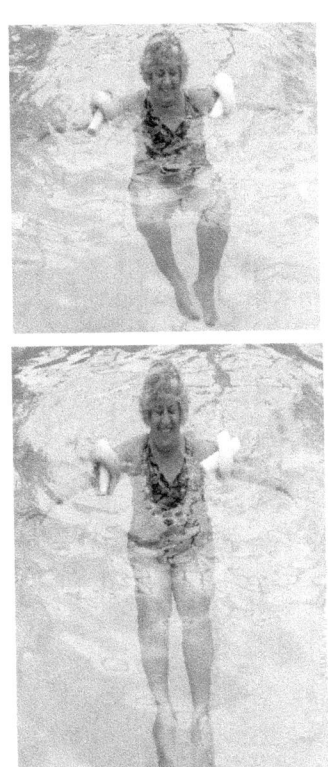

Knees in – Level One

Inhale and bring both knees towards your chest. As you exhale, push both feet away from your body. Continue bringing knees in towards your chest and pushing them away for at least eight repetitions.

Knees in - Level Two

Add speed to the movement. The faster you switch your legs, the harder and more intense the exercise will become. You can also add variety to the movement by fast and slower movements together.

Exercise Five:

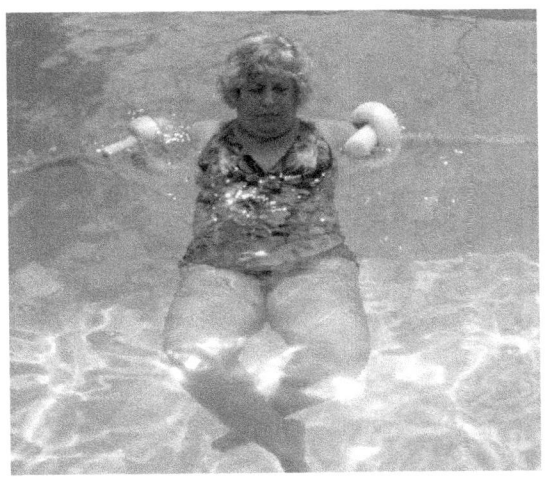

Cross your ankles and bring your knees up to your chest and back down to the starting position. Repeat for a total of eight repetitions.

You can also try bringing your legs behind you, and work them side to side.

Exercise Six:

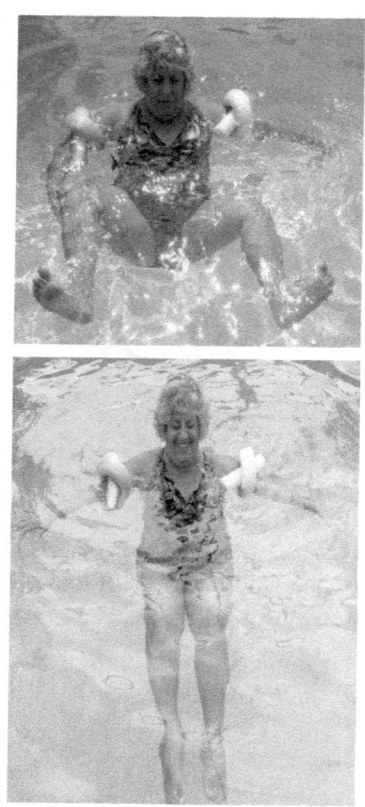

Knees in – Level One

Inhale and bring both knees out to your side and towards your chest. As you exhale, push both feet away from your body. Push through the heels of your feet. Keep your toes pointed upwards. Continue bringing knees in towards your chest and pushing them away for at least eight repetitions.

Knees in - Level Two

Add speed to the movement. The faster you switch your legs, the harder and more intense the exercise will become. You can also add variety to the movement by fast and slower movements together.

Exercise Seven:

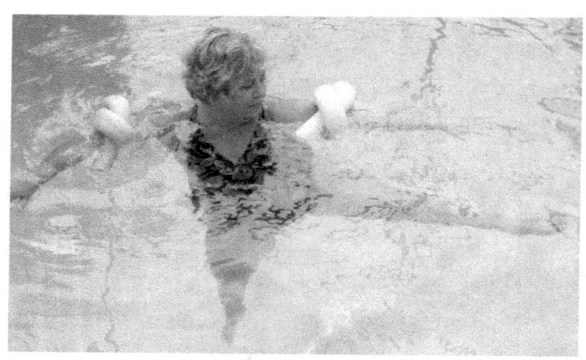

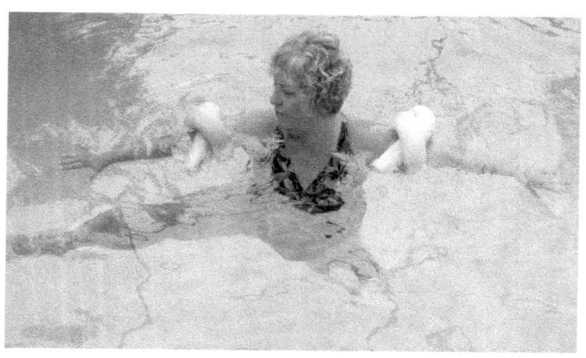

Level One

Inhale and as you exhale left ycur right leg out to your side as high up as you comfortably can. Repeat eight repetitions on your right side. When finished, repeat this exercise on your left leg.

Level Two

Add speed to your side leg lifts.

Level Three

Alternate your side leg lifts. You can speed in addition to alternating between the right and left legs.

Exercise Eight:

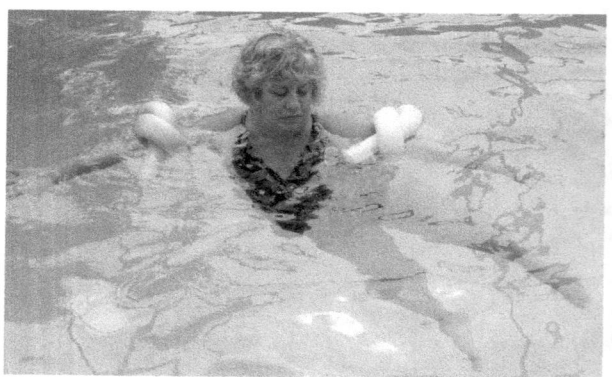

Keep your legs together and then bring them up to one side of your body, return to center, and bring them up to the other side. You can also do this exercise forward and backward and even make circles clockwise and counter-clockwise.

Exercise Nine:

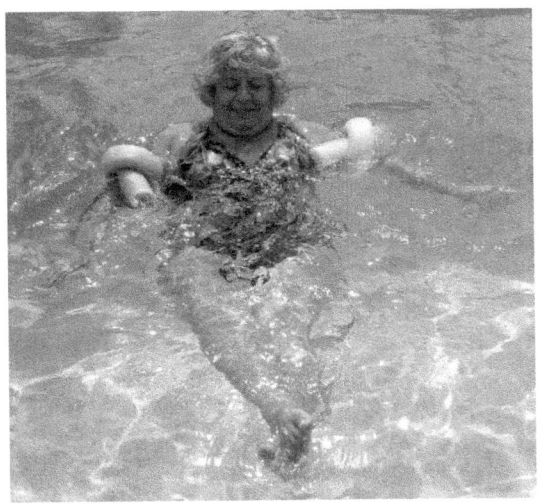

Bring your legs out in front of you and cross one foot over the other. Now twist your body from side to side. This is a great exercise for your core. Do for eight repetitions, then switch your feet and repeat for an additional eight repetitions.

Back, Buttocks and Legs

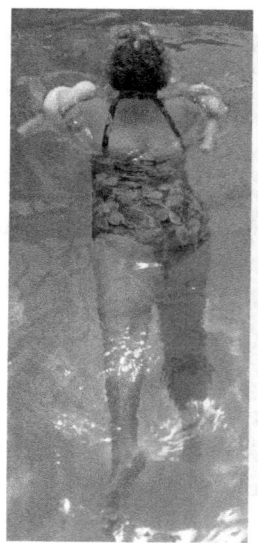 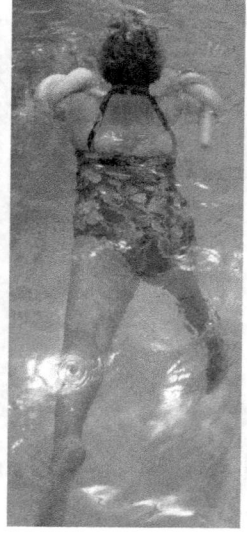

From the starting position bring one leg straight out behind you while you leave the other leg in the starting position. Repeat exercise with your other leg. Go as high up as you can with no back pain. Do eight repetitions for each leg.

Buttocks Kicks

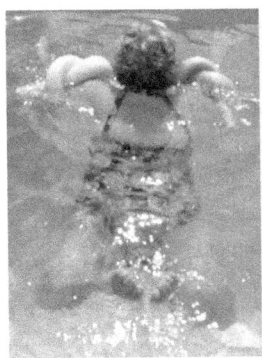 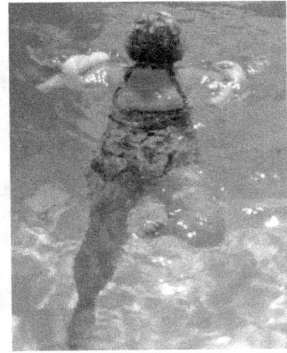

Bring both legs straight behind you. Alternate bringing the heel of one foot to your buttocks and release it. Do eight repetitions on one side and eight repetitions on the other side.

Now bring the heels of both of feet to your buttocks at the same time and release. Do eight repetitions.

Buttock Crossed Ankle Kicks

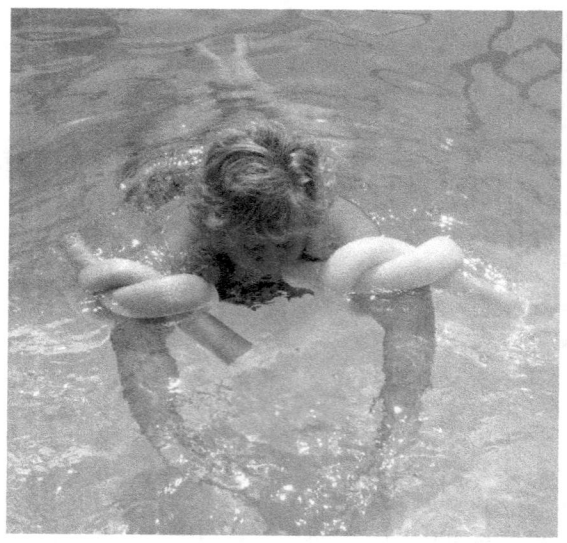

Cross your ankles and lean forward. Bring your feet to your buttocks and release. Do a total of eight repetitions. If this exercise hurts your back-then please stop doing it.

Abdominal Twists

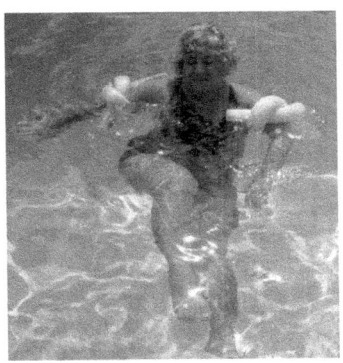

Level One-Inhale and bring both knees to your chest and as you exhale, twist your body, along with your knees to the right. Inhale and twist your body back to the center and as you exhale, twist to the other side. Repeat eight times.

Level Two-Repeat the same exercise as above only add speed to the twists. The faster you bring your knees in to your chest and back out, the more intense the workout will be.

Trim and Tone

Front Leg Lifts

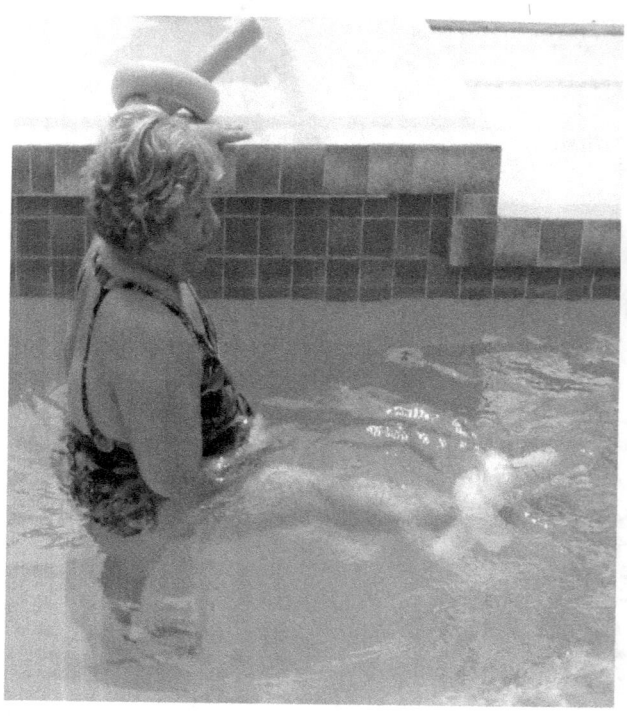

Level One-Begin with both feet planted firmly on the bottom of the pool and with your knees soft. Now, inhale and bring your left leg straight up in front of you as high as you comfortably can, hold for a few seconds, and then as exhale, bring your leg back down to the starting position. Repeat for a total of eight repetitions.

When finished, repeat the entire exercise with your right leg for a total of eight repetitions.

Level Two-Begin in the starting position listed above. This time you will alternate lifting your left leg and returning it to the starting position and then lifting your right leg and returning it to the starting position. Continue alternative the front leg lifts for a total of 16 repetitions.

Level Three-Repeat this exercise as listed in Level Two only add speed, hopping from right to left leg. You can also move forward and backward while alternating front leg lifts.

Side Leg Lifts

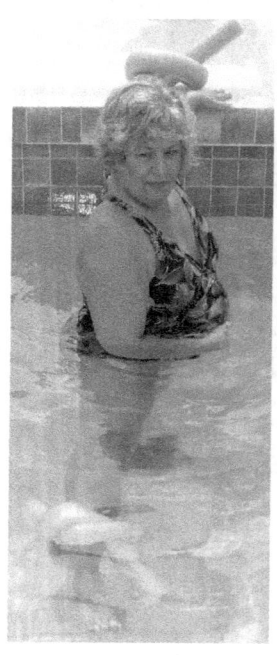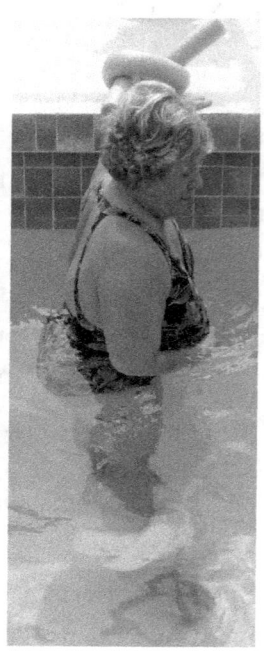

Level One-Plant both of your feet firmly on the bottom of the pool and keep your knees soft. Inhale and lift your right straight up at your side as high as you comfortably can, hold for a few seconds, and then exhale and release the leg back to the starting position. Repeat for a total of eight repetitions. Repeat the entire exercise on your left leg for a total of eight repetitions.

Level Two-Lift your right leg up as far as you can to your right side and return to the starting position. Then, lift your left leg up as far as you can to your left side and return to the starting position. Repeat alternating between the right leg and the left leg for a total of 16 repetitions.

Level Three-Add speed to the exercise shifting rapidly between the right and left leg lifts. You can also move forward and backward as you do this exercise. As an added treat, do this exercise while moving sideways from one end of the pool to the other. You can vary your speed and even add a double hop on one foot to add variety to your workout.

Back Leg Lifts

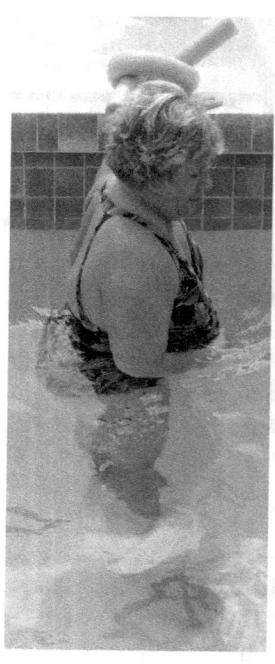 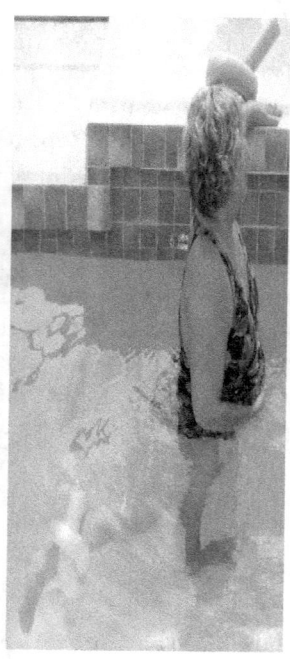

Back Leg Lifts – Level One

Begin with both feet planted firmly on the bottom of the pool and with your knees soft. Now, inhale and bring your left leg straight up behind you as high as you comfortably can, hold for a few seconds, and then as exhale, bring your leg back down to the starting position. Repeat for a total of eight repetitions. Repeat the entire exercise with your right leg for a total of eight repetitions.

Back Leg Lifts - Level Two

Alternate lifting your left and right leg behind you. Continue alternative the back leg lifts for a total of 16 repetitions.

Back Leg Lifts – Level Three

Repeat this exercise as listed in Level Two only add speed, hopping from right to left leg. You can also move forward and backward while alternating back leg lifts.

Hamstring Kicks

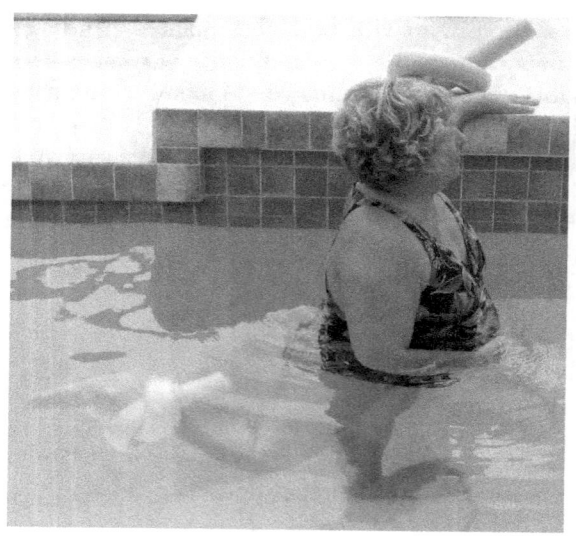

Begin with both feet planted firmly on the bottom of the pool and with your knees soft. Inhale and bring your left foot up to your buttocks, hold for a few seconds, and as exhale, bring your leg back down to the starting position. Repeat for a total of eight repetitions. Repeat your right leg for eight repetitions.

Shoulder Stretch

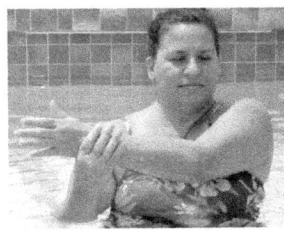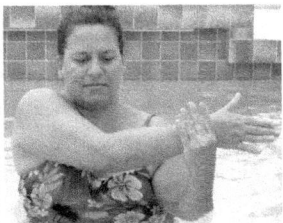

Begin the cool down by bring your straight left arm across the front of your body and gently grasp your left wrist with your right hand (as shown in picture #1). Gently press the left arm toward your right arm.

Be sure to keep your hips and body straight and looking forward. Do not force the stretch and be sure to inhale and exhale freely and easily. Release the arm.

Now, take your straight right arm and bring it across the front of your body and gently grasp your right wrist with your left hand and press the arms towards your left arm (as shown in picture #2). Release the arm. Repeat on both sides for an additional two more times.

Triceps Stretch

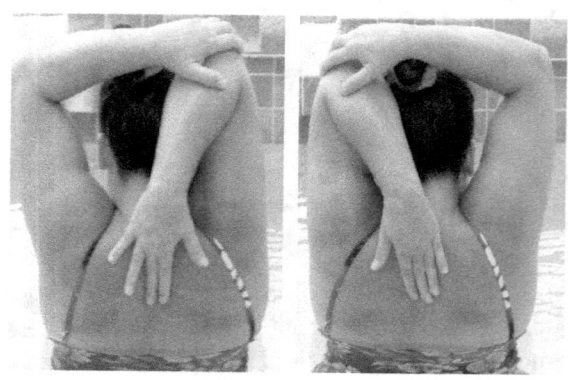

Bring your right arm straight out in front of your body and reach upward. Bend the elbow and bring the right hand down to lay flat on your back with the palm of your right hand on your back. Bring your left hand over and place it on your right elbow. Gently add pressure to your right elbow to push it backward giving you a stretch in your triceps muscle. Breathe normally.

Release and repeat on other arm.

4. Lat Stretch

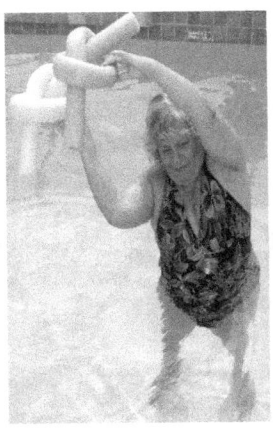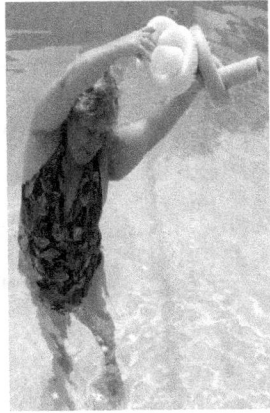

Inhale and reach both arms up over your head. Exhale, bend and reach your arms out to your right side, hold, inhale and return to center. Repeat stretching on to your left side. Do for a total of 16 repetitions.

Cool Down

Cool Downs are a series of movements that are used after an exercise class as a means to return the heart rate back to its normal pre-exercise rate. The more you exercise, the stronger your heart and lungs will become and the shorter the period of time it will take for the heart rate to return to normal. If you need help in adapting any of these exercises to your own specific limitations, just drop me an email at RevReikiND@cs.com and we can discuss options.

Cool Down

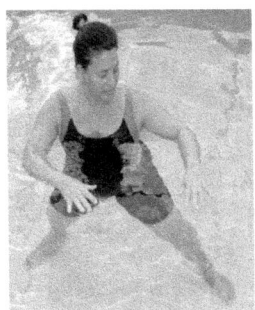 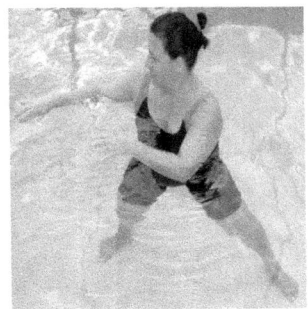

You can add mindfulness and Breath work to this cool down exercise. To do this exercise, spread your legs apart as far as you comfortably can to maintain your body's balance in the water.

Place your hands, palm down, at the very top of the water and pretend that there are flower petals floating on the top cf the water. Gently push the flower petals to the left and then to right trying not to disturb the petals, or the water.

About the Author

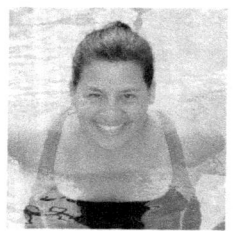

Francine Milford has Worked for more than 20 years in a variety of sports and exercise related classes, she is also an avid walker and enjoys reading a book audio tape while bicycling around the neighborhood.

A national and state licensed massage therapist and personal trainer, Francine has achieved certifications through the YMCA S.A.F.E. Aerobic Program, AEA Aquatics Exercise Association, ESA Exercise Safety Association, and AFAA Aerobics Fitness Association.

For more information and other book titles, visit: www.H2OWorkouts.com.